I0707069

This book is intended for educational purposes only. This book is not intended to diagnose, treat, or prescribe any skin treatments or products. Please see a professional skin therapist or dermatologist with any questions or concerns about your own skin conditions.

DEDICATION

To my husband Aaron, who endures endless lectures about all things science and skin care.

To my parents, for nurturing my love for science.

To my sister Sara, who shows me every day that anything is possible. You will always be my hero.

And most importantly, to all the other Estheticians on a quest for more information, there is nothing more valuable you can give yourself than the gift of knowledge.

<u>Special thanks to Hailey Rissolo for the cover design</u>

Table of Contents

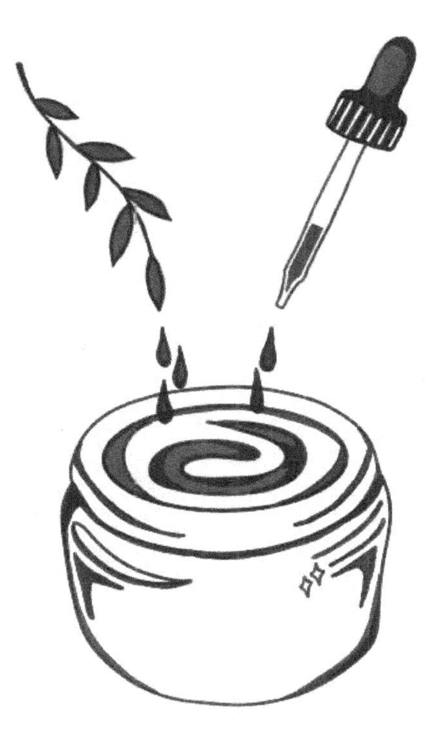

Chapter 1.

Introduction

In this book, I will review different ingredient types and their effect on the skin. The scientific area we are focusing on is biochemistry, sometimes called biological chemistry. Biochemistry is concentrating on the interactions between our cells and organic and inorganic molecules.

I feel that skin care ingredient science is a skimmed over topic in esthetics. After we are licensed, a lot of our ingredient knowledge comes from skincare company training, which in my experience is rushed over in order to get to the practical application. I am lucky enough that before I went to esthetician school, I received a bachelor's degree in biology, providing me with a deeper understanding of the chemical reactions and cellular changes that occur when we apply specific ingredients to the skin. However, working in the field, I saw a lot of my fellow Estheticians were missing that information. I wanted to be able to share my knowledge with other Estheticians, which inspired me to write this book.

As I explain types of ingredients, I will at times refer to the conclusions provided by scientific journal articles. Peer-reviewed scientific journal articles are the science community's standard for conveying and citing research findings. These articles have been reviewed and approved by a third party, removing the influence of bias. With my science background, this is the type of research I trust.

The goal of this book is to provide you a guide explaining the biochemistry behind these types of ingredients. When we understand the science of the

ingredient types, we increase our competency as licensed professionals. We are all striving to become masters of our craft, and a thorough understanding of the science behind skin care is another step on that path.

Chapter 2.

<u>The Consultation</u>

A quick word about consultations before we begin. The consultation is one of the most important parts of the facial service. Every client's skin is a puzzle, and you are the detective solving the mystery. During the consultation, ask what the current routine is, and look for gaps. Ask about previous treatments, any previous facials, chemical peels, or cosmetic procedures. Find out where they are from. I currently live in South Florida, and I can see it in the skin of the people who grew up down here (affectionately referred to as "Key West Skin").

When doing consultations, I aim to collect information that I refer to as ***The Three Factors of the***

<u>**Skin**</u>. The *first factor* is the skin we are born with (*our skin type*), the *second factor* is what our skin has been exposed to (*our environment, both in childhood and as an adult*) and the *third factor* is what we are currently doing to our skin (*the at-home skin care routine, facials, and any cosmetic procedures*).

When treating a client's skin, after receiving all three factors of information, we then can focus on the part we are in control of: *factor three. Factor three* is our skincare products and facial treatments, and more specifically, ***what type of ingredients are in those skincare products***. By understanding ingredient chemistry, you will be able to easily identify the appropriate services in the treatment room and products for each client's home care.

The success of skin improvement really depends on the esthetician's recommendations, so as licensed professionals we need to feel confident and well versed in ingredient types. By having this expertise, we will easily be able to identify the ingredient types and know exactly who this product would and would not be appropriate for.

This is a sample basic consultation that I use with all my new clients…

<u>Basic Consultation</u>

1. Primary skin concerns

2. Secondary skin concerns

3. Current skin routine

4. For men: any issues with shaving? Do you use a razor or buzzer?

5. Previous facials, chemical peels, laser treatments or other procedures? How were your results with those?

6. Allergies?

7. SPF daily?

8. Any cosmetics procedures in the last 2-3 weeks? Any cosmetic procedures scheduled for the future?

9. Any other medical conditions that would contraindicate you to receiving this treatment?

10. Any areas of the face, neck, chest, shoulders or arms I need to avoid?

Chapter 3

<u>Antioxidants</u>

We know antioxidants are good. We want them in our food and in our skincare. But why do we want them? <u>*And what exactly is an antioxidant?*</u>

From the Milady Standard Esthetics: Fundamentals (2012):

"Antioxidants prevent oxidation by neutralizing free radicals. Free radicals are super oxidizers that cause an oxidation reaction and produce a new free radical in the process. Because they are created by highly reactive atoms or molecules (often oxygen) free radicals are unstable. Left alone they will create inflammation, damage DNA, and eventually cause disease and death. One free radical can oxidize (combine or cause a substance to combine with oxygen)

millions of other substances. Antioxidants are free

radical scavengers that stop the oxidation reaction from

continuing" (page 170).

Okay, that is a lot of textbook-y words, let us

break it down a little bit.

"Antioxidants prevent oxidation by neutralizing

free radicals"

Okay, straight forward. But what is oxidation, a free

radical, and why do we want it neutralized?

"Free radicals are super oxidizers that cause an

oxidation reaction and produce a new free radical in the

process. Because they are created by highly reactive

atoms or molecules (often oxygen) free radicals are

unstable"

Okay, so free radicals are something that

interacts with other molecules to create an *oxidation*

reaction- which creates a NEW free radical, thus creating a chain reaction and an endless cycle of new free radical formation.

"Left alone they [free radicals] will create inflammation, damage DNA, and eventually cause disease and death"

Well now, these are terms we know. *Inflammation* in the cell means the cell must focus on repairing itself, and attention is taken away from normal healthy cell activity. All signs of aging and damaged skin come from inflammation. DNA is our genetic makeup, and we know DNA replicates itself. If our DNA gets damaged, the replicated copies will reflect that damage. So, these free radicals are bad guys, going in and messing things up within our cells.

"One free radical can oxidize (combine or cause a substance to combine with oxygen) millions of other substances"

This is the *OH CRAP* moment! One free radical can do the oxidation reaction (the one which damages the molecule it is interacting with and creates a new baby free radical in the process) and can do this process with MILLIONS OF SUBSTANCES. The potential for cell and tissue damage is unlimited.

Well, what the heck can we do? This is where our white knight hero comes into play….

Antioxidants are free radical scavengers that stop the oxidation reaction from continuing.

There is a solution to this unlimited potential damaging free radical bad guy…

<u>*Antioxidants!!*</u>

So now you understand what an antioxidant is: a white knight hero that swoops in and puts a stop to those pesky free radical bad guys that are causing limitless damage by stealing electrons, which in turn creates inflammation and DNA damage.

So, in summary, the next time a client asks you, "What do antioxidants actually do?" you are ready and confident to shell out a science packed answer! *"We need antioxidants in skincare because of those pesky free radicals' oxidizers and the endless potential for DNA damage and skin aging inflammation!"*

These are some of the most common antioxidants in the market today:

1. **<u>Vitamin C</u>**

     a. Magnesium Ascorbyl Phosphate (synthetic version)

     b. Ascorbic Acid or L-Ascorbic Acid (the most researched form)

Vitamin C is seen in anti-aging and hyperpigmentation targeting skin products because it has been shown in multiple studies to help prevent melanin formation and assist n collagen production. A few years ago, we saw this explosion of vitamin C products on the market because it is such an amazing and powerful antioxidant. However, vitamin C is unstable, degrades easily, and does not play well with others. Be mindful about combining vitamin C with other actives such as retinoids or acids.

Other forms that I haven't found a lot of research supporting its effectiveness one way or another include: **sodium ascorbyl phosphate, ascorbyl palmitate, tetrahexyldecyl ascorbate, magnesium ascorbyl phosphate, and ascorbyl glucoside**

2. <u>**Vitamin E**</u>

    a. Tocopherol

    b. Tocotrienols

Vitamin E has long been used for wounds and dry skin as it has been shown to promote skin healing. Vitamin E also works well with vitamin C, so you will often see them together. Vitamin E will stop free radicals, but in turn get damaged from the process. Vitamin C will repair the vitamin E and allow it to continue neutralizing the free radicals. Due to its wound healing properties, vitamin E is great for dry skin that requires nourishment.

3. **<u>Green Tea</u>**

    a. EGCG or Epigallocatechin gallate

Scientists have known green tea to be a powerful antioxidant when ingested, but it also works on the skin. Green tea works to regulate sebum production and has anti-inflammatory and anti-bacterial properties, which makes it an ideal ingredient for acne and sensitive skin.

4. **<u>Niacinamide</u>**

    a. Vitamin B3

    b. Nicotinic acid

Niacinamide is found naturally occurring within our bodies and in the food we eat. Niacinamide protects from free radical damage, repairs the skin barrier, and regulates oil production. It is great for all skin types, even acneic. Niacinamide can be used in conjunction with

vitamin A, vitamin C, retinols, or any other actives
without causing skin irritation.

5. **<u>Vitamin A</u>**

   I am going to cover a lot more about vitamin A/Retinoids in Chapter 5, but these are the forms of vitamin A that perform as antioxidants.

   a. Retinyl Ascorbate (A combination of vitamin A and vitamin C. By combining these two together they prove to be more stable).

   b. Retinyl Palmitate (A combination of vitamin A and palmitic acid. This compound is found naturally in our skin, working as an antioxidant, and protecting the skin from sun damage).

6. **<u>Resveratrol</u>**

    a. Polyphenol antioxidant

Resveratrol is found in grapes and berries and was a popular ingredient a few years ago. This ingredient is what these fruits use to protect themselves from infection and pollution. These attributes are what make it a good antioxidant, especially for acneic skin as it is naturally anti-bacterial and anti-inflammatory.

7. **<u>Coenzyme Q 10</u>**

    a. Ubiquinone

CoQ10 occurs naturally within our bodies, but like everything else, it decreases as we age making us prone to fine lines. This specific antioxidant helps stimulate collagen production, making it ideal for mature skin looking to minimize the appearance of fine lines and loss of elasticity.

Chapter 4

Stem Cells

I must admit something to you, my friend, nothing drives me crazier than a company boasting about their _plant stem cells_ in the magical serum that will fix everything. This is the ultimate tactic to grab the attention of the consumer with buzz words. I am going to break down the difference between _plant stem cells_ and _animal stem cells_, and what they are capable of.

Plant stem cells are going to be the ingredient you will most often see advertised. When I was early in my career as an Esthetician, I worked at a spa that carried a serum with apple stem cells. All the Estheticians loved it, singing its praises to the clients and each other. When I attended the training for this specific line, I was so excited to finally be able to ask the trainer, "How do plant stem cells work and communicate to our human (animal) cells?" I kid you not, this was her EXACT answer:

"Because plant stem cells are an organic ingredient, your body knows how to accept and work with this ingredient. Our bodies recognize things that are natural and organic and instinctively know how to process it."

I am sorry, but WHAT?! That is the biggest *"Let me just spew some BS because I have no idea, and no one has asked me this question before"* answer I had ever heard. I decided I would not accept that. So, I went on a hunt to find out more information about stem cells, and specifically, plant stem cells in skincare.

(This is probably the most science-heavy chapter in this book, but it needs to be. Stem cells are seriously deep biology, with many different aspects to them. I am

going to do my best to break this down into smaller

chunks.)

First, I am going to rew nd us back to high school biology class. There are two types of cells, **plant cells** and **animal cells**. These cells have a different biological makeup since plants and animals are in different kingdoms. Plant cells contain a cell wall, giving the cell a rigid structure, as well as chloroplast, which allows these organisms to make their own food from sunlight. Animal cells do not have a cell wall and require ingestion of an outside source to obtain nutrients. Cells are the basic structures of life, and when stripped down to their basic structures, animal cells and plant cells are like comparing a piece of steak to an apple.

So next we need to know what stem cells are exactly. In an article titled "Role of Cultured Skin

Fibroblasts in Aesthetic and Plastic Surgery" by Davood Mehrabani and Navid Manafi (2013), it is explained:

"Stem cells are unspecialized cells capable of renewing themselves through cell division without limit as long as the person is still alive. Each new cell has the potential either to remain a stem cell or become another type of cell"

Alright, now we are getting somewhere. Stem cells are a blank slate cell, with unlimited renewing potential to become a different type of cell.

But how does this relate to skin care?

At the 2018 *International Congress of Esthetics and Spa,* I attended a lecture by Daniel Cary, an Esthetician and honorary member of the Society of Cosmetic Chemists. I highly recommend attending any of his lectures as he is a wealth of knowledge when it comes to cosmetic chemistry. Daniel Cary explained stem cells' importance in terms of their role in skin care. Our cells are constantly communicating with each other, giving and receiving signals on what to do. These signals are messenger proteins referred to as *growth factors* and **we obtain these messenger proteins from stem cells**.

Now we are getting somewhere!

We now know what stem cells are and why we would want stem cells in skin care: **stem cells allow us to obtain the protein signals (*growth factors*) to ensure our skin cells are obtaining the messages to instruct them to work at their fullest potential.**

In reference to stem cells in skin care, we are most often referencing two types of animal adult stem cells:

1. **Adipose (Fat) Stem Cells**

2. **Bone Marrow Stem Cells***

*(*Information obtained from Daniel Cary's chapter in The Esthetician's Guide to Outstanding Esthetics Vol II (2018))*

(Note- **not included are *embryonic stem cells***. These cells are what receive a lot of buzz in the medical community and mainstream media for their ability to provide potential solutions to disease. However, for skin care purposes, these cells would not produce the growth factors needed to have an anti-inflammatory and wound healing effect.)

Have your eyes glazed over from this Cellular Biology lecture yet? I know, I am sorry I had to get very technical there, but it is important to **understand what animal stem cells do to understand what plant stem cells <u>cannot</u> do.**

Now for the most important sentence in this entire chapter, are you ready?

Plant stem cells do not produce the same protein growth factors as animal cells and therefore are <u>not</u> able to communicate with animal cells.

It is physically impossible to obtain the same results from plant stem cells in skin care that you would when using animal stem cells. Now, before we go trashing all the plant stem cell serums and moisturizers we have, plant stem cells do have some value in terms of skin care. Plant stem cells applied topically have been shown to act as antioxidants (and as we learned in Chapter 2, we love those!). Typically, we will see plant stem cells listed as a "cell culture" of either the swiss apple, argan fruit, grapes, or raspberry.

To summarize everything we just learned, there are benefits to animal stem cells in skin care, but not all stem cells are created equal, and plant stem cells should be viewed only as a fancy named antioxidant. (*Take that skin care line trainer who could not answer my question!*)

Want even more science? **(Because who does not want more science?!)**

For more information on:

Fibroblasts

Mehrabani, D., & Manafi, N. (2013). Role of cultured skin

fibroblasts in aesthetic and plastic surgery. _World

Journal of Plastic Surgery_, 2(1), 2–5.

Adipose Stem Cells

Miana, V. V., & González, E. (2018). Adipose tissue

stem cells in regenerative medicine.

Ecancermedicalscience, _12_, 822.

https://doi.org/10.3332/ecancer.2018.822

Bone Marrow Stem Cells

Fathke, C., Wilson, L., Hutter, J., Kapoor, V., Smith, A.,

Hocking, A., & Isik, F. (2004). Contribution of

bone marrow-derived cells to skin: collagen

deposition and wound repair. _Stem cells (Dayton,

Ohio)_, _22_(5), 812–822.

https://doi.org/10.1634/stemcells.22-5-812

Chapter 5

<u>Retinoids and Vitamin A</u>

When we talk about retinoids in skin care, we are talking about different forms of vitamin A ranging in strength. I want to beg n by defining the four types of retinoids we see in skincare:

1. **Retinoic Acid (RX only)** *A vitamin A derivative that has demonstrated an ability to alter collagen synthesis and is used to treat acne and visible signs of aging. Side effects are irritation, photosensitivity, skin dryness, redness, and peeling* (Milady Standard Esthetics: Fundamentals (2012), page 749).

   - Retinoic acid is the bioavailable form, meaning it is the form that your skin can readily use.

- Retinoic acid includes tretinoin (Retin-A), tazarotene (Tazorac), and adapalene (prescription-strength Differin).

2. **Retinol (Over the Counter)** *A natural form of vitamin A. It stimulates cell repair and helps to normalize skin cells by generating new cells* (Milady Standard Esthetics: Fundamentals (2012), page 749).

   - This includes anything you can buy without a doctor's prescription and will be listed as retinol in the ingredients list.

So those two we are familiar with, but there are two other categories of retinoids, the **esters**. This is where we branch into organic chemistry a little bit, but I am going to try to give you the simplest definition of an ester possible:

An ester is a compound derived from an acid, where hydrogen is replaced by a hydrocarbon.

To simplify this further, esters come from an acid, and they are a little different formula-wise. Since the formula is different from the original acid, esters are a weaker form of the acid. That is all that is important for us to know.

The two forms of vitamin A esters are:

1. **Retinoic Acid Esters** *These will be listed as Retinaldehyde or Granactive (hydroxypinacolone retinoate).*

2. **Retinyl/Retinol Esters** *I have seen the spelling both ways. These will be listed as Retinyl Propionate and Retinyl Palmitate*

So now that we know the four forms of retinoids, what is the difference between them all?

When applied topically, the skin must convert over the counter forms of retinoids into the bioavailable form (**retinoic acid**), by chemical conversion. Depending on the form of retinoid, it may require one, two, or three chemical reactions. Basic chemistry teaches us that when a compound goes through a chemical reaction, the strength of the compound weakens. So, we must know the form of retinoid we are utilizing to really know the strength. The other important factor to consider is that a weaker retinoid going through chemical conversions can be very irritating to the skin.

Weakest form to strongest form

Retinol Esters -> Retinol -> Retinoic Acid Esters -> Retinoic Acid

We must know this cycle so we can decipher percentages. For example, 1% retinol is weaker than

0.02% retinoic acid due to the chemical conversions it must go through.

Now that we know what to look for with vitamin A, let us look at **what happens in the skin**. Retinoids claim to increase collagen, lighten hyperpigmentation, and give an overall youthful appearance to the skin, but how is this happening?

Retinoids are considered ***keratolytic***, which means they encourage a quicker turnover of skin cells. This process allows for the sloughing off skin cells with hyperpigmentation. Retinoids also have properties that prevent new pigment from forming. In an article titled *"Depigmenting mechanisms of all-trans retinoic acid and retinol on B16 melanoma cells"*, Sato et al. (2008) found that the decrease in pigment from the use of retinoic acid and retinol was related to the inhibition of tyrosinase.

Therefore, we see hyperpigmentation decrease significantly over long-term use. Not only are the pigmented corneocytes being sloughed off, but also the pigment chemical reaction is being prevented from taking place. *(More about pigment production in Chapter 9).*

Retinoids also decrease the appearance of fine lines and wrinkles. In the article titled "*A comparative study of the effects of retinol and retinoic acid on histological, molecular, and clinic properties of human skin*" by Kong et al. (2016), an increase in epidermal thickness and collagen production was shown in the skin after four weeks of daily use of people who used either retinol or retinoic acid. This indicates that retinoids are stimulating the fibroblasts to produce more collagen and elastin.

In conclusion, retinoids work by exfoliating the corneocytes at an increased pace, increasing collagen production and preventing pigmentation. The type of retinoid selected makes a difference in the amount of these changes in the skin. Always encourage new retinol users to follow a slow and steady introduction. Remember, retinoids are the tortoise in the race. They will show improvements in the skin, but it requires patience.

<u>Articles Referenced</u>

Sato, K., Morita, M., Ichikawa, C., Takahashi, H., & Toriyama, M. (2008). Depigmenting mechanisms of all-trans retinoic acid and retinol on B16 melanoma cells. *Bioscience, Biotechnology, and Biochemistry, 72*(10), 2589–2597. doi: 10.1271/bbb.80279

Kong, R., Cui, Y., Fisher, G. J., Wang, X., Chen, Y., Schneider, L. M., & Majmudar, G. (2015). A comparative study of the effects of retinol and retinoic acid on histological, molecular, and clinical properties of human skin. *Journal of Cosmetic Dermatology, 15*(1), 49–57. doi: 10.1111/jocd.12193

Chapter 6

Peptides

We all love peptides. We tell our clients they are the "building blocks" of the skin and we need them to maintain the skin's structure. But what happens when we slather on those peptide-filled serums and moisturizers?

Milady Standard Esthetics: Fundamentals (2012) defines peptides as:

"Chains of amino acids that stimulate fibroblasts, cell metabolism, collagen, and improve skin's firmness. Larger chains are called polypeptides" (Page 746).

Okay, a quick breakdown of that definition:

- Fibroblasts are cells that create collagen and elastin.

- The **peptides** tell the fibroblasts to create more collagen and elastin.

- Collagen is a protein that not only gives skin its structure, but also promotes wound healing.

So, peptides stimulate our fibroblasts to make more collagen, thus leaving us with firm skin. Wound healing in terms of our skin refers more to the damage we receive from the sun, oxidative stress, and pollution, which break down the skin's structure. Peptides are organically found in every cell of our body. They keep our cells functioning properly, structured correctly, and receiving the important minerals they need.

When we refer to applying peptides topically onto the skin, we are typically referring to the activity of *signal peptides.* This type of peptide tricks our skin into thinking there has been an injury, thus promoting the wound healing process of creating more collagen.

However, there are a few other peptides that can be used in skin care. Specifically, *carrier peptides* deliver minerals to our skin to ensure the cells are functioning properly, *enzyme inhibitor peptides* slow down the skin's natural break down of collagen, and *neurotransmitter inhibiting peptides* block the chemicals that cause muscle contraction (resulting in the appearance of wrinkles).

Now all this sounds wonderful, but as estheticians, we must remember that topically applied ingredients have limitations. Peptides can support healthy skin, but they cannot change what the skin appears like genetically. In other words, peptides cannot do what cosmetic procedures can.

Let us talk for a moment about the names of peptides.

For example, *Palmitoyl Tripeptide-5*:

1. *Palmitoyl* is the name of the fatty acid connected to the peptide.

2. *Tripeptide* is the number of amino acids in the peptide (*Tri* meaning three).

3. And the number *5* is the length of the peptide.

Now, if all peptides were named this way it would not be too hard to decipher, but there is another way a peptide can be named. Peptides may also have the name a company has branded them, like *Matrixyl* (Palmitoyl Oligopeptide) or *Argeline* (Acetyl-Hexapeptide-8). Unfortunately, no matter how a peptide is named, the names do not tell you what type of peptide it is. For example, *Argeline* is a neurotransmitter inhibiting peptide, while *Matrixyl* is a signal peptide.

This is a copy of a table from an article by Schagen (2017). This article covers each of the peptides listed below and the supporting research to demonstrate the effectiveness. I highly recommend referring to the article for specific peptide information. This table does not include EVERY peptide on the market because not all peptides have documented controlled research performed supporting their efficacy. My advice when working with products with peptides is to ask your skincare rep for the studies on the specific peptide.

Signal Peptides	Carnosine, Copper tripeptide, Trifluoroacetyl-tripeptide-2, Tripeptide-10 citrulline, Acetyl tetrapeptide-5, Acetyl tetrapeptide-9, Acetyl tetrapeptide-11, Tetrapeptide PKEK, Tetrapeptide-21, Hexapeptide, Hexapeptide-11, Palmitoyl pentapeptide-4, Palmitoyl tripeptide-3/5, Palmitoyl tetrapeptide-7, Palmitoyl hexapeptide-12, Palmitoyl oligopeptide, Palmitoyl tripeptide-1, Pentamide-6
Carrier Peptides	Copper tripeptide, Manganese tripeptide-1
Neurotransmitter-inhibiting peptides	Acetyl hexapeptide-3, Pentapeptide-18, Pentapeptide-3, Tripeptide-3
Enzyme inhibitor peptides	Soybean peptide, Silk fibroin peptide, Black rice oligopeptide

Schagen, S. (2017). Topical Peptide Treatments with Effective Anti-Aging Results. *Cosmetics*, 4(2), 16. doi: 10.3390/cosmetics4020016

Chapter 7

<u>Ceramides</u>

Ceramides are popular ingredient types we often see in esthetics. They are usually found in moisturizers, serums, or cleansers. They are typically associated with anything meant to strengthen compromised skin.

The Milady Standard Esthetics: Fundamentals (2012) defines **ceramides** as:

"Glycolipid materials that are a natural part of the skin's intercellular matrix and barrier function" (Page 727).

In other words, ceramides are the *glycolipid* (naturally occurring long chains of lipids) component of *the intercellular matrix* (the stuff between the skin cells) and *barrier function* (the barrier that prevents trans-epidermal water loss).

There are a lot of ceramides on the market, and they usually have a name like *ceramide AP* or *ceramide NP*. Ceramides can either be organically derived from plants and animals or synthetically created. Organically derived ceramides are more often less stable or considered unethically produced by cruelty-free standards. Synthetic ceramides have come a long way since original formulation and do a great job.

The claims of a product containing ceramides are referring to what happens when the skin is reinforced with ceramides as opposed to what the ceramides do. By repairing the skin's barrier and reinforcing the intercellular matrix with ceramides, the skin will appear and act healthy, feel hydrated and supple, and have less appearance of fine lines.

Ceramides, like most other things our bodies naturally produce, decrease production as we age. This is a type of ingredient we would want to integrate into home care for a client with mature skin or compromised barrier function in need of soothing and strengthening.

Chapter 8

Enzymes

Within the skin, the natural process of shedding corneocytes slows down with age and sometimes needs a little extra help. When these corneocytes do not shed naturally, they stick together and become like glue. This can create a wide range of conditions on the skin like acne, texture, dehydration, and dull appearance. To combat these conditions, we can use enzymes.

So, what are enzymes and how do they exfoliate our skin?

Enzymes are organic molecules, found within all living things. Enzymes are referred to as a catalyst, as they increase the rate of chemical reactions without undergoing any damage. What this means is the enzyme can assist in multiple chemical reactions in a row without being damaged. There are different types of enzymes that specialize in different processes. In skin care we are usually referring to *proteolytic enzymes.*

Proteolytic enzymes specialize in the breakdown of the protein bonds that cause the older corneocytes to stick together. The breakdown of these protein bonds results in an acceleration in the sloughing of corneocytes. The encouraged removal of these cells is why after using enzymes the skin is left with a brighter appearance. The other benefit of using enzymes is that they leave the skin more readily available to perform extractions and to absorb serums and moisturizers.

In skin care we will find enzymes in the treatment room and in-home care exfoliants. Some enzyme products claim to be gentle enough to be used every day, but this really depends on the client's skin. The two common enzymes we see in esthetics are papaya (papin, papaya proteinase), and pineapple (bromelain, sulfhydryl proteases). I have seen pumpkin enzymes advertised, but I am unable to find a supporting scientific journal article about the effectiveness and stability supporting the use of pumpkin enzymes.

In summary, enzymes are a great ingredient when combating certain skin concerns, such as dullness and dehydration. The gentle surface level exfoliation enzymes provide allows us to use this beneficial ingredient on a multitude of skin types and conditions.

For a very in-depth explanation on enzymes:

Robinson, P. K. (2015). Enzymes: Principles and biotechnological applications. *Essays in Biochemistry, 59*, 1–41. https://doi.org/10.1042/bse0590001

Chapter 10

<u>Tyrosinase Inhibitors</u>

Another ingredient that requires consistency and patience is tyrosinase inhibitors. Tyrosinase inhibitors should be incorporated in home care for clients whose concerns are hyperpigmentation. To fully understand tyrosinase inhibitors, we first need to be clear about where the excess pigment on skin comes from.

Let us define a couple of terms first.

From Milady Standard Esthetics: Fundamentals (2012):

"***Melanocytes****: cells that produce skin pigment granules in the basal layer*" (Page 742).

"*Melanosomes: pigment carrying granules*" (Page 236).

"*Melanin: tiny grains of pigment (coloring matter) that are produced by melanocytes and deposited into cells in that stratum germinativum layer of the epidermis*" (Page 742).

To put it all together...

Melanocytes are cells that produce pigment granules (**melanosomes**), which then carry and produce a protein called **melanin,** which is transferred from the **melanosomes** into the keratinocytes.

This process is known as **melanogenesis**.

So now we know how melanin is produced in the skin, but what about when melanin is produced to create an uneven skin tone, sunspots, or acne scars? When trauma occurs to our skin in the form of an acne pustule, sun exposure, or other damaging external factors, inflammation is created in the skin. Inflammation signals to our melanocytes to produce extra pigment as a form of protection for the skin. This chemical process of pigment creation can also be seen when you cut an apple in half and leave it on the counter for a few hours. The browning of the apple is caused by something called tyrosinase. This is the same enzyme in our skin creating uneven brown pigment.

According to Milady Standard Esthetics: Fundamentals (2012):

*"**Tyrosinase** is an enzyme that converts tyrosine, an amino acid, into melanin"* (Page 316).

Tyrosinase is an enzyme (see Chapter 8) responsible for starting the chemical reaction that leads to the production of melanin. A way for us to combat melanogenesis is by utlizing ingredients that stop tyrosinase, known as **tyrosinase inhibitors.** When helping a client with pigmentation issues of the skin, it is not enough to exfoliate the pigmented cells at the surface- the root of the problem must be addressed as well. Tyrosinase inhibitors allow us to slow or stop the melanogenesis cycle, targeting the origin of the pigmentation chemical reaction.

Common Tyrosinase Inhibitors

1. Kojic Acid

    - A by-product of Japanese rice wine.

2. Azelaic Acid-/ Dicarboxylic acid

    - Derived from grains like barley, wheat, and rye, or created synthetically.

3. Vitamin C / L-ascorbic acid

   - Naturally derived or synthetically created, the efficacy depends on the formulation, the stabilizers, and product packaging.

4. Hydroquinone

   - A long-time gold standard for treating hyperpigmentation with a lot of controversy. This ingredient is legal in The United States and can be bought over the counter or by prescription.

5. Licorice Root Extract/ Glabridin

   - Studies suggest this to be more effective than kojic acid and ascorbic acid as a tyrosinase inhibitor.

6. Bearberry/ Arbutin

   - Can be synthetic or naturally derived, seen as an alternative to hydroquinone.

7. Retinoids (See Chapter 5 on Retinoids and Vitamin A).

This is a small list, but there are tons of different ingredients being tested all the time for the efficacy as a tyrosinase inhibitor. Always look for scientific studies supporting the claims of any new ingredient.

<u>Additional information on Tyrosinase Inhibitors</u>

Zolghadri, S., Bahrami, A., Hassan Khan, M. T., Munoz-Munoz, J., Garcia-Molina, F., Garcia-Canovas, F., & Saboury, A. A. (2019). A comprehensive review on tyrosinase inhibitors. *Journal of Enzyme Inhibition and Medicinal Chemistry, 34*(1), 279–309. https://doi.org/10.1080/14756366.2018.1545767

Pillaiyar, T., Manickam, M., & Namasivayam, V. (2017). Skin whitening agents: Medicinal chemistry perspective of tyrosinase inhibitors. *Journal of Enzyme Inhibition and Medicinal Chemistry, 32*(1), 403–425. https://doi.org/10.1080/14756366.2016.1256882

Chapter 10

<u>Facial Oils</u>

I am a firm believer in the ability of a facial oil to change the skin. Facial oils can provide nourishment to the skin in a way that may be missing from moisturizers. Try to think of the skin as a person with the basic needs of food, water, and shelter. To me, facial oils are the food for the skin. (Serums being the water and moisturizer and SPF being the shelter).

Facial oils are usually derived from seeds or nuts of different plants. In every seed, there are nutrients used to nurture it while it grows into a plant. Every seed has a different combination of nutrients for that specific plant, which is why it is important to know the properties of the more common facial oils. I have created a cheat sheet with some facts about popular facial oils and which skin types would benefit from them.

A quick word about *oleic acid* and *linoleic acid* before we get started.

__*Linoleic acid*__ is a polyunsaturated omega-6 essential fatty acid, which means it is necessary for humans and animals to have, but we cannot synthesize it on our own (we must ingest it). *Linoleic acid* is found in many plant oils in different amounts. The amazing thing about *linoleic acid* is that it has been shown in laboratory studies to inhibit melanin production when applied to the skin by reducing tyrosinase activity.

On the other hand, __*oleic acid*__ is a monounsaturated omega-9 non-essential fatty acid, meaning it occurs organically in the fats of animals or vegetable oils. *Oleic acid* is most often associated with olive oil. You can feel when the oil is high in *oleic acid* as it is not quick to absorb into the skin, with a heavy occlusive consistency. *Oleic acid* can disrupt the skin's barrier or be irritating to the skin. However, due to its skin barrier disrupting properties, *oleic acid* can assist in product penetration.

Facial Oil Cheat Sheet

1. Jojoba Oil

All Skin Types

    a. From the seed of the jojoba plant, *Simmondsia chinensis*

    b. Helps regulate sebum production

    c. Deeply moisturizing

    d. Anti-inflammatory

    e. 5% Linoleic acid and 5-15% Oleic acid *

2. Rosehip Oil

Oily/Mature Skin

    a. From the seeds of the wild rose bush, *Rosa moschata* or *Rosa rubiginosa*

    b. Regulates sebum production in the skin

    c. Anti-inflammatory

    d. 44% Linoleic ac d and 13.9% Oleic acid *

3. Squalane Oil

All Skin Types

    a. Formally extracted from sharks, but is now manufactured from sugar cane

    b. A non-greasy, richer emollient version of our skin's own natural oil (sebum is made up partly of squalane)

    c. Replenishes and restores our lipid barrier

    d. *Squalene* is the oxidized version of squalane, which can trigger acne.

4. Grape Seed Oil

Oily/Acneic

    a. An oil from the seeds of grapes

    b. Regulates sebum production

    c. Rich antioxidants

    d. Anti-inflammatory

    e. Inhibits melanin formation

    f. 70% Linoleic acid and 16% Oleic acid *

5. Sea Buckthorn Oil

Mature/ Dry

   a. From the Sea buckthorn, *Hippophae rhamnoides*, it can be extracted from either the pulp of the berries or the seeds

   b. Rich in antioxidants

   c. 6% Linoleic acid and 28% Oleic acid * (*Note, this oil has a different % of Linoleic and Oleic acid depending on if the oil is from the fruit or the seeds, or a combination of the two*)

6. Marula Oil

Mature/Dry

   a. Comes from the nuts of the Marula tree

   b. Used as a moisturizing agent in Africa for years

   c. Rich in antioxidants

   d. 7% Linoleic acid and 78% Oleic acid *

7. Sunflower Seed Oil / Sunflower Oil

Dry

   a. From sunflower seeds

   b. Usually a carrier oil for other ingredients

   c. 14-40% Linoleic acid and 48-74%Oleic

       acid *

8. Safflower Seed Oil

Mature/ Dry/ Sensitive

   a. Extracted from the seeds of a flowering

       plant, *Carthamus tinctorius*

   b. Anti-inflammatory

   c. Melanin inhibiting

   d. 68-83% Linoleic Acid and 8-21% Oleic

       acid*

9. Argan Oil

Dehydrated/Dry

   a. From the kernels of the argan tree,

       sometimes referred to as Moroccan oil as it

       is unique to Morocco

b. Improves skin elasticity, hydration, and

barrier function

c. Can be used to prevent ingrown hairs

d. 29-36% Linoleic acid and 43-49% Oleic

acid*

*Percentages of Linoleic acid and Oleic acid were obtained from Lab Muffin's website, a skin ingredient educator with a Chemistry PhD.

The percentages vary due to the source of the plant, and the method of creation.

https://labmuffin.com/why-linoleic-acid-and-rosehip-oil-might-fix-your-skin/

Chapter 11

<u>AHAs,BHAs, LHAs, and PHAs</u>

I do not think I need to spend too much time on this chapter. I feel this is the one area of Esthetics school where there is a good amount of focus. I am just going to do a brief run-down of the different chemical exfoliants and how they work. At the end of this chapter I will also cover some lesser talked about chemical exfoliants.

Alpha hydroxy acids are defined by Milady Standard Esthetics: Fundamentals (2012) as:

"Acids derived from plants (mostly fruit) that are often used to exfoliate the skin; mild acids; glycolic, lactic, malic, and tartaric acid. AHAs exfoliate by loosening the bonds between dead corneum cells and

dissolve the intracellular matrix. Alpha hydroxy acids also stimulate cell renewal" (Page 723).

What this is telling us is that alpha hydroxy acids (derived either naturally or synthetically) break down the bonds between the skin cells, thus encouraging the sloughing off these corneocytes. Doing so reveals younger more refined skin that appears much smoother, is more hydrated, and, over time, becomes visibly firmer.

AHA's, Smallest to Largest

Glycolic acid: Comes from sugarcane and is the smallest AHA with the deepest penetration. Specifically known for its ability to retexturize skin.

Lactic acid: Found in foods that go through a bacteria fermentation process (sour milk, pickles, beer).

Lactic acid is also a great moisturizing ingredient due to increasing the water holding ability of the skin.

Malic acid: Found naturally occurring in apples and cherries, it is the third smallest of the AHA's. I find this acid is rarely used by itself, but instead is found in conjunction with other AHA's.

Tartaric acid: Found in red wine, it is also an antioxidant. This acid is more often used to stabilize the pH for other AHA's.

Citric acid: From citrus fruits, this acid is typically used more as a pH adjuster in a product as opposed to an actual exfoliant. The pH of citric acid is around 2.2, which makes it very irritating to the skin in large percentages.

Mandelic acid: Derived from bitter almonds and is the largest of the AHA's. This AHA is a good choice for sensitive and dry skin as the penetration of the product is limited and research has shown that this ingredient may increase sebum production.

On the other hand, we have **_beta hydroxy acids_**, which essentially refers to salicylic acid. The Milady Standard Esthetics: Fundamentals (2012) defines BHA's as:

"Beta hydroxy acids (BHAs), exfoliating organic acid; salicylic acid; milder than alpha hydroxy acids (AHAs). BHAs dissolve oil and are beneficial for oily skin" (page 725).

The last sentence of that definition is the most important part of BHAs. Due to its ability to dissolve oil, salicylic acid enters the pore, loosening the dead skin cells and oil that build up within the pore. Salicylic acid is derived from the willow bark or birch tree, which gives it antimicrobial and antiseptic benefits. Another great benefit of salicylic acid is its ability to calm and soothe irritated skin.

PHAs or *polyhydroxy acids* are like AHAs in that they dissolve the bonds that hold the corneocytes together but are limited by their large size. Examples of PHAs are gluconolactone, galactose, and lactobionic acid. PHAs are often found in skincare products in combination with AHAs as they work nicely together to exfoliate, brighten, and hydrate the skin.

LHAs or *lipohydroxy acids* work along the skin's surface by detaching the bonds between individual corneocytes as well as decreasing the bacteria within the pores. LHAs are a much larger molecule then BHAS and AHAS, so it is well tolerated by sensitive skin. Within skincare products you may see LHAs listed as *capryloyl salicylic acid* as it is a derivative of salicylic acid. A great article by Dr. Joshua Zeichner* discusses studies showing LHAs making a significant reduction in acne pustules and an improvement in skin tone and smoothness. LHAs have also been shown to increase collagen and elastin production like the use of tretinoin.

For more information on the research done, I recommend reading the entire article:

Zeichner J. A. (2016). The Use of Lipohydroxy Acid in Skin Care and Acne Treatment. *The Journal of clinical and aesthetic dermatology*, 9(11), 40–43.

Chapter 12

<u>Conclusion</u>

There are a lot of false claims in the skincare industry these days. You will see the hottest new ingredient everywhere, followed by promises of how it will change the skin. No one will provide you with the knowledge you need to see through certain false claims- that duty falls into your hands. You are responsible for seeing through the smoke and mirrors to know how the skin is impacted by specific ingredient types.

I hope this book provided you with knowledge of biochemistry and the confidence to speak on these concepts. To be respected as skincare specialists, every piece of information we can gain will increase our value and expertise to better serve our clients.

My final hope is that you will share this education with your Esthetician peers. The best gift we can give ourselves and each other is knowledge. When we spread knowledge to our skin specialist peers, we further the professional image of the Esthetician community.

<u># Great Resources for Skin Care Ingredient Chemistry and Biology</u>

Clary, D. (2018). *Estheticians Guide to Outstanding Esthetics (Volumes I and II)*. Createspace.

Gerson, J., DAngelo, J. M., Deitz, S., & Lotz, S. (2012). *Milady standard esthetics: fundamentals (11th ed.)*. Clifton Park, NY: Cengage Learning.

Lab Muffin Beauty Science, a skin ingredient educator with a Chemistry PhD.
https://labmuffin.com/

Michalun, N., & Michalun, M. V. (2014). *Miladys skin care and cosmetic ingredients dictionary*. Australia: Delmar.

Nerida Joy, with over 40 years in the skin care field, she is an Esthetician I really admire. She provides education to estheticians as she works with real clients on her YouTube and offers classes on her website.
https://educateyourskin.com/

Paula's Choice Skincare Ingredient Dictionary
https://www.paulaschoice.com/ingredient-dictionary

US National Library of Medicine National Institutes of Health.
(PubMed Central)
https://www.ncbi.nlm.nih.gov/pmc/

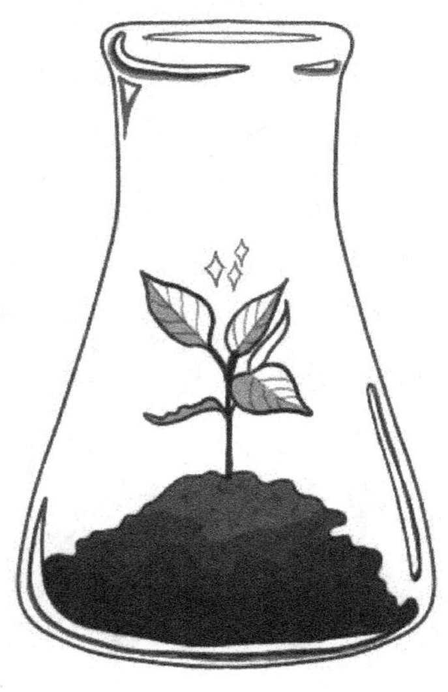